The *Family* Medical Journal

Get it together

Dianne Terry

Réalta Publications

Publshed by Réalta Publications in 2019

First Edition; First printing

Design and writing by Dianne Terry

ISBN: 978-0-9600417-8-7

This Journal belongs to

____

If found, please call

____

In Case of Emergency, please contact

____

____

Dedication

This book is dedicated to my family. Being a mom and grandmother is a precious gift, one I don't take lightly.

Table of Contents

A Personal Note to You

Life is busy. As moms and dads, we have so many things that take up our time just keeping life on track—being a breadwinner, parent, chauffeur, homework-checker, cook, bedtime-story-reader, nurse . . . the list goes on and on. We get so busy, sometimes the little stuff—the papers that need to be organized, for example—can slip through the cracks.

My hope is you will use this journal on a regular basis to help you get it together—capture all the medical information for every member of your family in one place.

How to Use This Journal

1. Fill out the important information at the front of this journal as soon as you can. You will find this a handy guide.
2. Medical Insurance. Fill out your insurance information. In addition to your primary and secondary insurance, you may have cancer insurance, and other types of supplemental health insurance as well.
3. Members of your family. You know who they are.
4. For each member of the family, there will be a group of pages containing important health information including
   - Blood type, allergies, medical alert info, surgeries and serious injuries
   - Illnesses/conditions, family history
   - Doctors and hospitals used by each member—since that information can vary
   - Medications—both prescriptions and over the counter
   - Immunization records
5. There's also a section for 25 office visits.
6. You may find it helpful to color coordinate each person's section in the journal. Then you can tie the office visit to a family member by color-coding it as well.

Calendar

Year: ________

Monday	Tuesday	Wednesday
☐	☐	☐
☐	☐	☐
☐	☐	☐
☐	☐	☐
☐	☐	☐

Notes: ____________________

Calendar

Month: ________________

Thursday	Friday	Saturday / Sunday
☐	☐	☐ ☐
☐	☐	☐ ☐
☐	☐	☐ ☐
☐	☐	☐ ☐
☐	☐	☐ ☐

Notes: ________________

Calendar

Year: ________

Monday	Tuesday	Wednesday
☐	☐	☐
☐	☐	☐
☐	☐	☐
☐	☐	☐
☐	☐	☐

Notes: ____________________

Calendar

Month: ______________

Thursday	Friday	Saturday / Sunday
☐	☐	☐ ☐
☐	☐	☐ ☐
☐	☐	☐ ☐
☐	☐	☐ ☐
☐	☐	☐ ☐

Notes: ____

Calendar

Year: ________

Monday	Tuesday	Wednesday

Notes: ______________________________

Calendar

Year: ________

Monday	Tuesday	Wednesday
☐	☐	☐
☐	☐	☐
☐	☐	☐
☐	☐	☐
☐	☐	☐

Notes: ____

Calendar

Year: ________

Monday	Tuesday	Wednesday
☐	☐	☐
☐	☐	☐
☐	☐	☐
☐	☐	☐
☐	☐	☐

Notes: ________________________________

Month: ______________

Calendar

Thursday	Friday	Saturday / Sunday
☐	☐	☐ / ☐
☐	☐	☐ / ☐
☐	☐	☐ / ☐
☐	☐	☐ / ☐
☐	☐	☐ / ☐

Notes: ____

Calendar

Year: ________

Monday	Tuesday	Wednesday
☐	☐	☐
☐	☐	☐
☐	☐	☐
☐	☐	☐
☐	☐	☐

Notes: ________________________________

Calendar

Month: ____________

Thursday	Friday	Saturday / Sunday
☐	☐	☐ / ☐
☐	☐	☐ / ☐
☐	☐	☐ / ☐
☐	☐	☐ / ☐
☐	☐	☐ / ☐

Notes: ____________

Calendar

Year: ________

Monday	Tuesday	Wednesday
☐	☐	☐
☐	☐	☐
☐	☐	☐
☐	☐	☐
☐	☐	☐

Notes: ________________________________

Calendar

Month: ________________

Thursday	Friday	Saturday / Sunday
☐	☐	☐ ☐
☐	☐	☐ ☐
☐	☐	☐ ☐
☐	☐	☐ ☐
☐	☐	☐ ☐

Notes: ____________________

Calendar

Year: ____________

Monday	Tuesday	Wednesday
☐	☐	☐
☐	☐	☐
☐	☐	☐
☐	☐	☐
☐	☐	☐

Notes: ____

Calendar

Month: ______________

Thursday	Friday	Saturday / Sunday
☐	☐	☐ / ☐
☐	☐	☐ / ☐
☐	☐	☐ / ☐
☐	☐	☐ / ☐
☐	☐	☐ / ☐

Notes: ______________________________

____

____

____

____

Calendar

Year: ________

Monday	Tuesday	Wednesday
☐	☐	☐
☐	☐	☐
☐	☐	☐
☐	☐	☐
☐	☐	☐

Notes: ____________________

Month: ______________

Calendar

Thursday	Friday	Saturday / Sunday
☐	☐	☐ / ☐
☐	☐	☐ / ☐
☐	☐	☐ / ☐
☐	☐	☐ / ☐
☐	☐	☐ / ☐

Notes: ____

Calendar

Year: ________

Monday	Tuesday	Wednesday
☐	☐	☐
☐	☐	☐
☐	☐	☐
☐	☐	☐
☐	☐	☐

Notes: ____________________

Calendar

Month: ______________

Thursday	Friday	Saturday / Sunday
☐	☐	☐ / ☐
☐	☐	☐ / ☐
☐	☐	☐ / ☐
☐	☐	☐ / ☐
☐	☐	☐ / ☐

Notes: ____

Calendar

Year: ________

Monday	Tuesday	Wednesday
☐	☐	☐
☐	☐	☐
☐	☐	☐
☐	☐	☐
☐	☐	☐

Notes: ________________________________

Calendar

Month: ______________

Thursday	Friday	Saturday / Sunday

Notes: ____________________

Calendar

Year: ________

Monday	Tuesday	Wednesday
☐	☐	☐
☐	☐	☐
☐	☐	☐
☐	☐	☐
☐	☐	☐

Notes: ____

____

____

____

____

Calendar

Month: ______________

Thursday	Friday	Saturday / Sunday
☐	☐	☐ Saturday ☐ Sunday
☐	☐	☐ ☐
☐	☐	☐ ☐
☐	☐	☐ ☐
☐	☐	☐ ☐

Notes: ____

Calendar

Year: ________

Monday	Tuesday	Wednesday
☐	☐	☐
☐	☐	☐
☐	☐	☐
☐	☐	☐
☐	☐	☐

Notes: ____

____

____

____

____

Calendar

Month: ______________

Thursday	Friday	Saturday / Sunday

Notes: ____________________

Medical Insurance

Primary Insurance: ______________________________
Policy #: ______________________________
Policy Start Date:______________ **Policy End Date:**______________
Address: ______________________________
City/State/Zip: ______________________________
____
Contact: ______________________________
Phone: ______________________________
Email:______________________________

Secondary Insurance: ______________________________
Policy #: ______________________________
Policy Start Date:______________ **Policy End Date:**______________
Address: ______________________________
City/State/Zip: ______________________________
____
Contact: ______________________________
Phone: ______________________________
Email:______________________________

Additional Insurance: ______________________________
Policy #: ______________________________
Policy Start Date:______________ **Policy End Date:**______________
Address: ______________________________
City/State/Zip: ______________________________
____
Contact: ______________________________
Phone: ______________________________
Email:______________________________

Additional Insurance: ______________________________
Policy #: ______________________________
Policy Start Date:______________ **Policy End Date:**______________
Address: ______________________________
City/State/Zip: ______________________________
____
Contact: ______________________________
Phone: ______________________________
Email:______________________________

Additional Medical Insurance

Additional Insurance: ______________________________
Policy #: ______________________________
Policy Start Date:________________ **Policy End Date:**________________
Address: ______________________________
City/State/Zip: ______________________________
____
Contact: ______________________________
Phone: ______________________________
Email:______________________________

Additional Insurance: ______________________________
Policy #: ______________________________
Policy Start Date:________________ **Policy End Date:**________________
Address: ______________________________
City/State/Zip: ______________________________
____
Contact: ______________________________
Phone: ______________________________
Email:______________________________

Additional Insurance: ______________________________
Policy #: ______________________________
Policy Start Date:________________ **Policy End Date:**________________
Address: ______________________________
City/State/Zip: ______________________________
____
Contact: ______________________________
Phone: ______________________________
Email:______________________________

Additional Insurance: ______________________________
Policy #: ______________________________
Policy Start Date:________________ **Policy End Date:**________________
Address: ______________________________
City/State/Zip: ______________________________
____
Contact: ______________________________
Phone: ______________________________
Email:______________________________

Members of our family

Dad

Name: ____

Birthdate: ______________________ Age: _______________

Mom

Name: ____

Birthdate: ______________________ Age: _______________

Child 1

Name: ____

Birthdate: ______________________ Age: _______________

Child 2

Name: ____

Birthdate: ______________________ Age: _______________

Child 3

Name: ____

Birthdate: ______________________ Age: _______________

Child 4

Name: ____

Birthdate: ______________________ Age: _______________

Child 5

Name: ____

Birthdate: ______________________ Age: _______________

Dad's Medical Info

Blood Type: ______________________

Allergies: ____

____

____

____

Medical Alert Information: ______________________________

____

____

____

____

Previous Surgeries:

Date: ______________ **Surgeon:** ____________________

Surgery: ____

____

____

Date: ______________ **Surgeon:** ____________________

Surgery: ____

____

____

Date: ______________ **Surgeon:** ____________________

Surgery: ____

____

____

Date: ______________ **Surgeon:** ____________________

Surgery: ____

____

____

Date: ______________ **Surgeon:** ____________________

Surgery: ____

____

____

Serious Injuries:

Date: ____________________ **Surgeon:** ____

Injury: ____

____

____

Date: ____________________ **Surgeon:** ____

Injury: ____

____

____

Date: ____________________ **Surgeon:** ____

Injury: ____

____

____

Date: ____________________ **Surgeon:** ____

Injury: ____

____

____

Date: ____________________ **Surgeon:** ____

Injury: ____

____

____

NOTES:

Dad's Personal Medical History

	Rheumatic Fever		Lung (Pulmonary Disease)
	Heart Disease		COPD
	Heart Attack >50		Water on the Lungs
	Heart Attack <50		Asthma
	High Blood Pressure		Type I Diabetes
	AFib—Atrial Fibrillation		Type II Diabetes
	Pacemaker		Type III Diabetes
	Heart Murmur		Hepatitis A, B, or C
	High Cholesterol		Headaches/Migraines (w/aura)
	Stroke		Headaches/Migraines (w/out aura)
	Whooping Cough (Pertussis)		Seizure Disorder
	Measles		Epilepsy
	Meningitis		Digestive Tract
	Chicken Pox (Varicella)		Gallbladder/Gallstones
	Mumps		Diabetes
	Pneumonia		Liver Disease / Hepatitis
	Polio		Thyroid
	Tuberculosis		Kidney Renal Disease
	HIV Infection		Kidney Stones
	Eczema		Prostate Problems
	Tattoo		Rheumatoid Arthritis
	Hay Fever		Prior Orthopedic Problems
	Hives (Uticaria)		Joint Problems
	Allergies		Depression / Suicide
	Ear/Nose/Throat		Alcoholism
	Hearing Problems		Drug Addiction
	Immune Disorder		Anxiety

Dad's Personal Medical History (cont'd)

	Skin Cancer		Panic Attacks
	Cancer		Mental Health Disorder
	Anemia		Fertility
	Hernia: Type ______________		Colon Polyps? ____
			Type: __________________

Dad's Family Medical History

Condition	* G/A/U C/P/S	Condition	* G/A/U C/P/S
Heart Disease		Cancer	
Heart Attack		Breast	
High Blood Pressure		Colorectal	
High Cholesterol		Lung	
Kidney Disease		Prostate / Ovarian	
Lung Disease		Skin	
Asthma		Other: _____________	
COPD		Liver Disease	
Migraines		Stroke	
Dementia		Tuberculosis	
Alzheimers		Depression/Suicide	
Mental Disorder		Epilepsy/Seizures	
Thyroid Disease		Diabetes	
Smokers		Alcoholism	
Osteoporosis		Drug Addiction	

*** G/A/U/C/P/S = Grandparent, Aunt, Uncle, Cousin, Parent, Sibling**

Dad's Doctors and Hospitals

HOSPITAL: ______________________________

Address: ______________________________

____

City/State/Zip: ______________________________

____

Phone: ______________________________

Fax: ______________________________

PRIMARY CARE: ______________________________

Address: ______________________________

____

City/State/Zip: ______________________________

____

Phone: ______________________________

Fax: ______________________________

DENTIST: ______________________________

Address: ______________________________

____

City/State/Zip: ______________________________

____

Phone: ______________________________

Fax: ______________________________

OPTOMETRIST: ______________________________

Address: ______________________________

____

City/State/Zip: ______________________________

____

Phone: ______________________________

Fax: ______________________________

SPECIALIST: ______________________________

Address: ______________________________

____

City/State/Zip: ______________________________

____

Phone: ______________________________

Fax: ______________________________

Dad's Doctors and Hospitals

SPECIALIST: ______________________________

Address:______________________________

____

City/State/Zip:______________________________

____

Phone:______________________________

Fax:______________________________

SPECIALIST: ______________________________

Address:______________________________

____

City/State/Zip:______________________________

____

Phone:______________________________

Fax:______________________________

SPECIALIST: ______________________________

Address:______________________________

____

City/State/Zip:______________________________

____

Phone:______________________________

Fax:______________________________

SPECIALIST: ______________________________

Address:______________________________

____

City/State/Zip:______________________________

____

Phone:______________________________

Fax:______________________________

SPECIALIST: ______________________________

Address:______________________________

____

City/State/Zip:______________________________

____

Phone:______________________________

Fax:______________________________

Dad's Medications

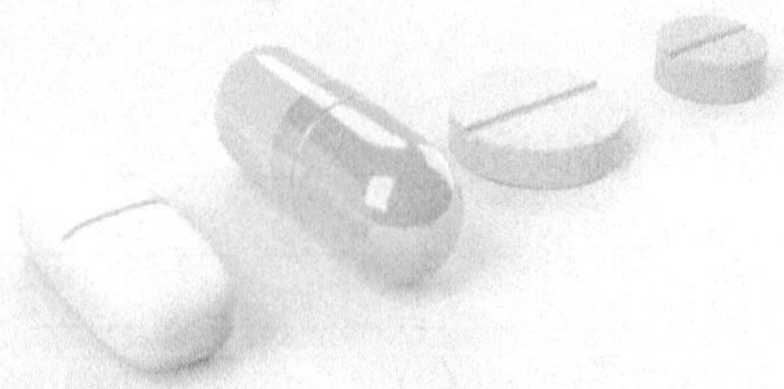

Prescriptions

Name	Dosage	Frequency	What's it For?

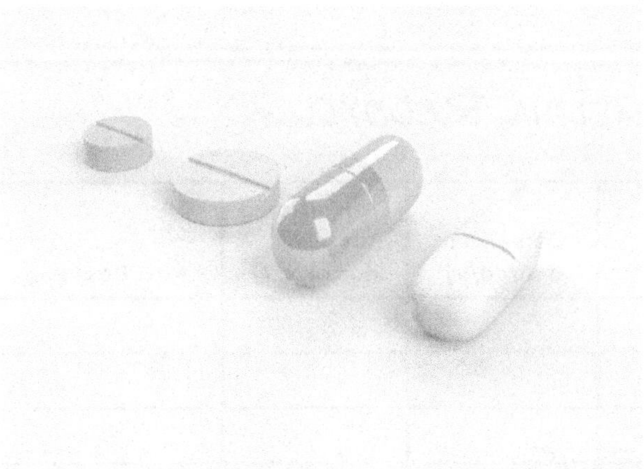

Dad's Medications

Vitamins and Supplements

Name	Dosage	Frequency	What's it For?

Dad's Immunization Record

Vaccine	Type	Date Given (mm/dd/yy)	Administered by (clinic, doctor, etc)	Next Dose Date
Diptheria, Tetanus, Pertusis (e.g. Tdap, Td)				
Hepatitis A				
Hepatitis B				
Human Pappilomavirus				
Measles, Mumps, Rubella				
Varicella (Checkenpox)				
Meningococcal ACWY				
Meningococcal B				
Pneumococcal conjugate				
Pneumococcal polysacharide				
Hib				

Dad's Immunization Record (cont'd)

Vaccine	Type	Date Given (mm/dd/yy)	Administered by (clinic, doctor, etc)	Next Dose Date
Influenza				
Zoster (shingles)				

How to Complete this Record

1. With the exception of hepatitis B vaccines, record the generic abbreviation (e.g., Tdap) or the trade name for each vaccine; for hepatitis B vaccines, record the trade name (see table at right).
2. Record the type of vaccine (i.e. HepA-HepB)
3. Record the date given.
4. Record the source of the vaccine given (clinic, doctor, etc.).
5. Record when the next dose is due if necessary.

Mom's Medical Info

Blood Type: ______________________

Allergies: ____

____

____

____

Medical Alert Information: ______________________________

____

____

____

____

Previous Surgeries:

Date: ______________ **Surgeon:** ____________________

Surgery: ____

____

____

Date: ______________ **Surgeon:** ____________________

Surgery: ____

____

____

Date: ______________ **Surgeon:** ____________________

Surgery: ____

____

____

Date: ______________ **Surgeon:** ____________________

Surgery: ____

____

____

Date: ______________ **Surgeon:** ____________________

Surgery: ____

____

____

Serious Injuries:

Date: ____________________ **Surgeon:** ______________________________________
Injury: ____
____
____

Date: ____________________ **Surgeon:** ______________________________________
Injury: ____
____
____

Date: ____________________ **Surgeon:** ______________________________________
Injury: ____
____
____

Date: ____________________ **Surgeon:** ______________________________________
Injury: ____
____
____

Date: ____________________ **Surgeon:** ______________________________________
Injury: ____
____
____

NOTES:

Mom's Personal Medical History

	Rheumatic Fever		Lung (Pulmonary Disease)
	Heart Disease		COPD
	Heart Attack >50		Water on the Lungs
	Heart Attack <50		Asthma
	High Blood Pressure		Type I Diabetes
	AFib—Atrial Fibrillation		Type II Diabetes
	Pacemaker		Type III Diabetes
	Heart Murmur		Hepatitis A, B, or C
	High Cholesterol		Headaches/Migraines (w/aura)
	Stroke		Headaches/Migraines (w/out aura)
	Whooping Cough (Pertussis)		Seizure Disorder
	Measles		Epilepsy
	Meningitis		Digestive Tract
	Chicken Pox (Varicella)		Gallbladder/Gallstones
	Mumps		Diabetes
	Pneumonia		Liver Disease / Hepatitis
	Polio		Thyroid
	Tuberculosis		Kidney Renal Disease
	HIV Infection		Kidney Stones
	Eczema		Prostate Problems
	Tattoo		Rheumatoid Arthritis
	Hay Fever		Prior Orthopedic Problems
	Hives (Uticaria)		Joint Problems
	Allergies		Depression / Suicide
	Ear/Nose/Throat		Alcoholism
	Hearing Problems		Drug Addiction
	Immune Disorder		Anxiety

Mom's Personal Medical History (cont'd)

	Skin Cancer		Panic Attacks
	Cancer		Mental Health Disorder
	Anemia		Fertility
	Hernia: Type _______________		Colon Polyps? ____
			Type: ___________________

Mom's Family Medical History

Condition	* G/A/U C/P/S	Condition	* G/A/U C/P/S
Heart Disease		Cancer	
Heart Attack		Breast	
High Blood Pressure		Colorectal	
High Cholesterol		Lung	
Kidney Disease		Prostate / Ovarian	
Lung Disease		Skin	
Asthma		Other: _____________	
COPD		Liver Disease	
Migraines		Stroke	
Dementia		Tuberculosis	
Alzheimers		Depression/Suicide	
Mental Disorder		Epilepsy/Seizures	
Thyroid Disease		Diabetes	
Smokers		Alcoholism	
Osteoporosis		Drug Addiction	

*** G/A/U/C/P/S = Grandparent, Aunt, Uncle, Cousin, Parent, Sibling**

Mom's Doctors and Hospitals

HOSPITAL: ______________________________
Address:______________________________
____
City/State/Zip:______________________________
____
Phone:______________________________
Fax:______________________________

PRIMARY CARE: ______________________________
Address:______________________________
____
City/State/Zip:______________________________
____
Phone:______________________________
Fax:______________________________

DENTIST: ______________________________
Address:______________________________
____
City/State/Zip:______________________________
____
Phone:______________________________
Fax:______________________________

OPTOMETRIST: ______________________________
Address:______________________________
____
City/State/Zip:______________________________
____
Phone:______________________________
Fax:______________________________

SPECIALIST: ______________________________
Address:______________________________
____
City/State/Zip:______________________________
____
Phone:______________________________
Fax:______________________________

Mom's Doctors and Hospitals

SPECIALIST: ______________________________
Address:______________________________
____
City/State/Zip:______________________________
____
Phone:______________________________
Fax:______________________________

SPECIALIST: ______________________________
Address:______________________________
____
City/State/Zip:______________________________
____
Phone:______________________________
Fax:______________________________

SPECIALIST: ______________________________
Address:______________________________
____
City/State/Zip:______________________________
____
Phone:______________________________
Fax:______________________________

SPECIALIST: ______________________________
Address:______________________________
____
City/State/Zip:______________________________
____
Phone:______________________________
Fax:______________________________

SPECIALIST: ______________________________
Address:______________________________
____
City/State/Zip:______________________________
____
Phone:______________________________
Fax:______________________________

Mom's Medications

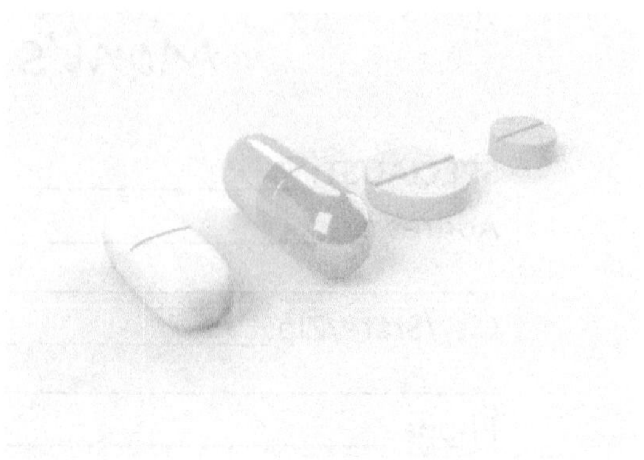

Prescriptions

Name	Dosage	Frequency	What's it For?

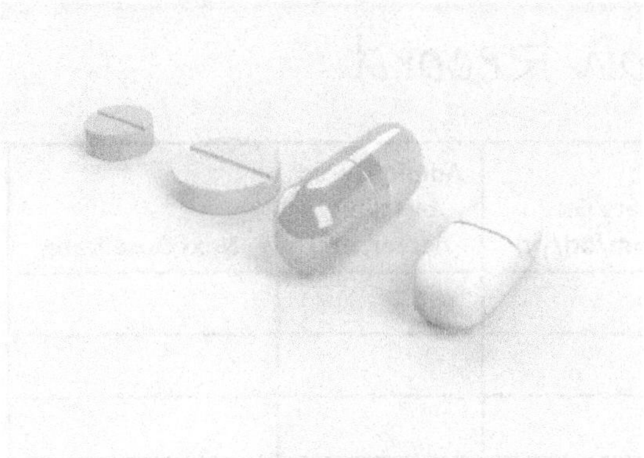

Mom's Medications

Vitamins and Supplements

Name	Dosage	Frequency	What's it For?

Mom's Immunization Record

Vaccine	Type	Date Given (mm/dd/yy)	Administered by (clinic, doctor, etc)	Next Dose Date
Diptheria, Tetanus, Pertusis (e.g. Tdap, Td)				
Hepatitis A				
Hepatitis B				
Human Pappilomavirus				
Measles, Mumps, Rubella				
Varicella (Checkenpox)				
Meningococcal ACWY				
Meningococcal B				
Pneumococcal conjugate				
Pneumococcal polysacharide				
Hib				

Mom's Immunization Record (cont'd)

Vaccine	Type	Date Given (mm/dd/yy)	Administered by (clinic, doctor, etc)	Next Dose Date
Influenza				
Zoster (shingles)				

How to Complete this Record

1. With the exception of hepatitis B vaccines, record the generic abbreviation (e.g., Tdap) or the trade name for each vaccine; for hepatitis B vaccines, record the trade name (see table at right).
2. Record the type of vaccine (i.e. HepA-HepB)
3. Record the date given.
4. Record the source of the vaccine given (clinic, doctor, etc.).
5. Record when the next dose is due if necessary.

____________ Medical Info

Blood Type: ____________________

Allergies: ____

____

____

____

Medical Alert Information: ______________________________

____

____

____

____

Previous Surgeries:

Date: ____________ **Surgeon:** ______________________

Surgery: ____

____

____

Date: ____________ **Surgeon:** ______________________

Surgery: ____

____

____

Date: ____________ **Surgeon:** ______________________

Surgery: ____

____

____

Date: ____________ **Surgeon:** ______________________

Surgery: ____

____

____

Date: ____________ **Surgeon:** ______________________

Surgery: ____

____

____

Serious Injuries:

Date: ____________________ **Surgeon:** ____

Injury: ____

____

____

Date: ____________________ **Surgeon:** ____

Injury: ____

____

____

Date: ____________________ **Surgeon:** ____

Injury: ____

____

____

Date: ____________________ **Surgeon:** ____

Injury: ____

____

____

Date: ____________________ **Surgeon:** ____

Injury: ____

____

____

NOTES:

_______________ Personal Medical History

	Rheumatic Fever		Lung (Pulmonary Disease)
	Heart Disease		COPD
	Heart Attack >50		Water on the Lungs
	Heart Attack <50		Asthma
	High Blood Pressure		Type I Diabetes
	AFib—Atrial Fibrillation		Type II Diabetes
	Pacemaker		Type III Diabetes
	Heart Murmur		Hepatitis A, B, or C
	High Cholesterol		Headaches/Migraines (w/aura)
	Stroke		Headaches/Migraines (w/out aura)
	Whooping Cough (Pertussis)		Seizure Disorder
	Measles		Epilepsy
	Meningitis		Digestive Tract
	Chicken Pox (Varicella)		Gallbladder/Gallstones
	Mumps		Diabetes
	Pneumonia		Liver Disease / Hepatitis
	Polio		Thyroid
	Tuberculosis		Kidney Renal Disease
	HIV Infection		Kidney Stones
	Eczema		Prostate Problems
	Tattoo		Rheumatoid Arthritis
	Hay Fever		Prior Orthopedic Problems
	Hives (Uticaria)		Joint Problems
	Allergies		Depression / Suicide
	Ear/Nose/Throat		Alcoholism
	Hearing Problems		Drug Addiction
	Immune Disorder		Anxiety

____________ Personal Medical History (cont'd)

	Skin Cancer		Panic Attacks
	Cancer		Mental Health Disorder
	Anemia		Fertility
	Hernia: Type ______________		Colon Polyps? ____
			Type: __________________

____________ Family Medical History

Condition	* G/A/U C/P/S	Condition	* G/A/U C/P/S
Heart Disease		Cancer	
Heart Attack		Breast	
High Blood Pressure		Colorectal	
High Cholesterol		Lung	
Kidney Disease		Prostate / Ovarian	
Lung Disease		Skin	
Asthma		Other: ____________	
COPD		Liver Disease	
Migraines		Stroke	
Dementia		Tuberculosis	
Alzheimers		Depression/Suicide	
Mental Disorder		Epilepsy/Seizures	
Thyroid Disease		Diabetes	
Smokers		Alcoholism	
Osteoporosis		Drug Addiction	

*** G/A/U/C/P/S = Grandparent, Aunt, Uncle, Cousin, Parent, Sibling**

________Doctors and Hospitals

HOSPITAL: ______________________________
Address:______________________________
____
City/State/Zip:______________________________
____
Phone:______________________________
Fax:______________________________

PRIMARY CARE: ______________________________
Address:______________________________
____
City/State/Zip:______________________________
____
Phone:______________________________
Fax:______________________________

DENTIST: ______________________________
Address:______________________________
____
City/State/Zip:______________________________
____
Phone:______________________________
Fax:______________________________

OPTOMETRIST: ______________________________
Address:______________________________
____
City/State/Zip:______________________________
____
Phone:______________________________
Fax:______________________________

SPECIALIST: ______________________________
Address:______________________________
____
City/State/Zip:______________________________
____
Phone:______________________________
Fax:______________________________

__________Doctors and Hospitals

SPECIALIST: ______________________________
Address:______________________________
____
City/State/Zip:______________________________
____
Phone:______________________________
Fax:______________________________

SPECIALIST: ______________________________
Address:______________________________
____
City/State/Zip:______________________________
____
Phone:______________________________
Fax:______________________________

SPECIALIST: ______________________________
Address:______________________________
____
City/State/Zip:______________________________
____
Phone:______________________________
Fax:______________________________

SPECIALIST: ______________________________
Address:______________________________
____
City/State/Zip:______________________________
____
Phone:______________________________
Fax:______________________________

SPECIALIST: ______________________________
Address:______________________________
____
City/State/Zip:______________________________
____
Phone:______________________________
Fax:______________________________

______________Medications

Prescriptions

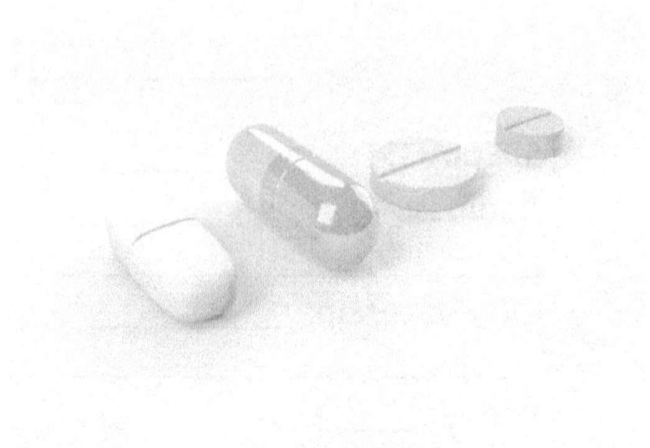

Name	Dosage	Frequency	What's it For?

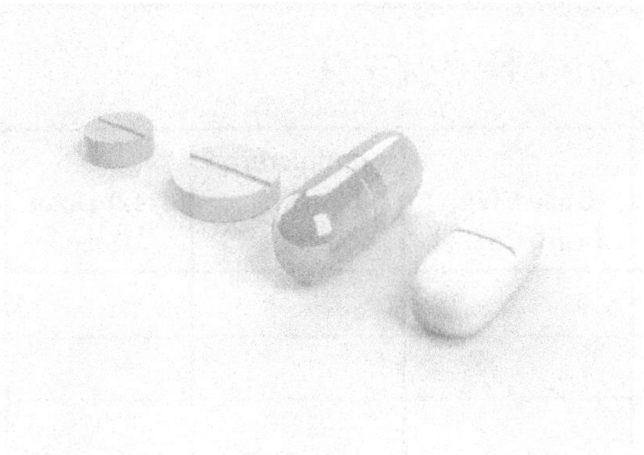

______________Medications

Vitamins and Supplements

Name	Dosage	Frequency	What's it For?

____________ Immunization Record

Vaccine	Type	Date Given (mm/dd/yy)	Administered by (clinic, doctor, etc)	Next Dose Date
Hepatitis B				
Rotavirus				
Diptheria, Tetanus, Pertusis (e.g. Tdap, Td)				
Haemophilus influenzae type b (Hib)				
Pneumococcal conjugate				
Inactivated poliovirus				

Immunization Record (cont'd)

Vaccine	Type	Date Given (mm/dd/yy)	Administered by (clinic, doctor, etc)	Next Dose Date
Influenza				
Measles, Mumps, Rubella				
Varicella (Checkenpox)				

______________ Immunization Record

Vaccine	Type	Date Given (mm/dd/yy)	Administered by (clinic, doc-tor, etc)	Next Dose Date
Hepatitis A				
Meningococcal ACWY				
Tetanus, diptheria, & acellular pertussis				
Human Pappilomavirus				
Meningococcal B				
Pneumococcal polysacharide				

How to Complete this Record

1. With the exception of hepatitis B vaccines, record the generic abbreviation (e.g., Tdap) or

   the trade name for each vaccine; for hepatitis B vaccines, record the trade name .
2. Record the type of vaccine (i.e. HepA-HepB)
3. Record the date given.
4. Record the source of the vaccine given (clinic, doctor, etc.).
5. Record when the next dose is due if necessary.

Immunization Record (cont'd)

Immunization information:

Diphtheria, tetanus, and pertussis (DTaP)

Routine vacc: 5-dose series at 2, 4, 6, 15-18 months, 4-6 years

Haemophilus influenzae type b vaccination

Routine vacc:

ActHIB, Hiberix, or Pentacel: 4-dose series at 2, 4, 6, 12-15 mos

PedvaxHIB: 3-dose series at 2, 4, 12-15 months

Hepatitis A

Routine vacc:—2-dose series

Hepatitis B

Routine vacc: 3 dose series at 0, 1-2, 6-18 months

Human papillomavirus vaccination

2– or 3-dose series depending on age at initial vaccination

Inactivated poliovirus vaccination

Routine vacc: 4-dose series at ages 2, 4, 6-18 mos, 4-6 yrs

Influenza vaccination

Routine vacc: 1 dose any influenza vaccine - annually

Measles, mumps, and rubella

Routine vacc: 2-dose series at 12-15 months, 4-6 years

Meningococcal ACWY

Routine vacc: 2-dose series: 11-12 years, 16 years

Pneumococcal vaccination

Routine vacc: 4-dose series at 2, 4, 6, 12-15 months

Rotavirus vaccination

Routine vacc:

Rotarix: 2-dose series at 2 and 4 months

RotaTeq: 3-dose series at 2, 4, and 6 months

Tetanus, diphtheria, and pertussis (Tdap) vaccination

Routine vaccination: Adolescents age 11-12 years—1 dose Tdap

Varicella vaccination

Routine vaccination: 2-dose series: 12-15 months, 4-6 years

________________Medical Info

Blood Type: ____________________________

Allergies: ____

____

____

____

Medical Alert Information:____

____

____

____

____

Previous Surgeries:

Date: ___________________ **Surgeon:** ____________________________________

Surgery: ____

____

____

Date: ___________________ **Surgeon:** ____________________________________

Surgery: ____

____

____

Date: ___________________ **Surgeon:** ____________________________________

Surgery: ____

____

____

Date: ___________________ **Surgeon:** ____________________________________

Surgery: ____

____

____

Date: ___________________ **Surgeon:** ____________________________________

Surgery: ____

____

____

Serious Injuries:

Date: ____________________ **Surgeon:** ______________________________________

Injury: ____

____

____

Date: ____________________ **Surgeon:** ______________________________________

Injury: ____

____

____

Date: ____________________ **Surgeon:** ______________________________________

Injury: ____

____

____

Date: ____________________ **Surgeon:** ______________________________________

Injury: ____

____

____

Date: ____________________ **Surgeon:** ______________________________________

Injury: ____

____

____

NOTES:

____________ Personal Medical History

	Rheumatic Fever		Lung (Pulmonary Disease)
	Heart Disease		COPD
	Heart Attack >50		Water on the Lungs
	Heart Attack <50		Asthma
	High Blood Pressure		Type I Diabetes
	AFib—Atrial Fibrillation		Type II Diabetes
	Pacemaker		Type III Diabetes
	Heart Murmur		Hepatitis A, B, or C
	High Cholesterol		Headaches/Migraines (w/aura)
	Stroke		Headaches/Migraines (w/out aura)
	Whooping Cough (Pertussis)		Seizure Disorder
	Measles		Epilepsy
	Meningitis		Digestive Tract
	Chicken Pox (Varicella)		Gallbladder/Gallstones
	Mumps		Diabetes
	Pneumonia		Liver Disease / Hepatitis
	Polio		Thyroid
	Tuberculosis		Kidney Renal Disease
	HIV Infection		Kidney Stones
	Eczema		Prostate Problems
	Tattoo		Rheumatoid Arthritis
	Hay Fever		Prior Orthopedic Problems
	Hives (Uticaria)		Joint Problems
	Allergies		Depression / Suicide
	Ear/Nose/Throat		Alcoholism
	Hearing Problems		Drug Addiction
	Immune Disorder		Anxiety

____________ Personal Medical History (cont'd)

	Skin Cancer		Panic Attacks
	Cancer		Mental Health Disorder
	Anemia		Fertility
	Hernia: Type _______________		Colon Polyps? ____
			Type: ____________________

____________ Family Medical History

Condition	* G/A/U C/P/S	Condition	* G/A/U C/P/S
Heart Disease		Cancer	
Heart Attack		Breast	
High Blood Pressure		Colorectal	
High Cholesterol		Lung	
Kidney Disease		Prostate / Ovarian	
Lung Disease		Skin	
Asthma		Other: _____________	
COPD		Liver Disease	
Migraines		Stroke	
Dementia		Tuberculosis	
Alzheimers		Depression/Suicide	
Mental Disorder		Epilepsy/Seizures	
Thyroid Disease		Diabetes	
Smokers		Alcoholism	
Osteoporosis		Drug Addiction	

*** G/A/U/C/P/S = Grandparent, Aunt, Uncle, Cousin, Parent, Sibling**

__________Doctors and Hospitals

HOSPITAL: ____
Address:____
____
City/State/Zip:____
____
Phone:____
Fax:____

PRIMARY CARE: ____
Address:____
____
City/State/Zip:____
____
Phone:____
Fax:____

DENTIST: ____
Address:____
____
City/State/Zip:____
____
Phone:____
Fax:____

OPTOMETRIST: ____
Address:____
____
City/State/Zip:____
____
Phone:____
Fax:____

SPECIALIST: ____
Address:____
____
City/State/Zip:____
____
Phone:____
Fax:____

________Doctors and Hospitals

SPECIALIST: ______________________________
Address:______________________________
____
City/State/Zip:______________________________
____
Phone:______________________________
Fax:______________________________

SPECIALIST: ______________________________
Address:______________________________
____
City/State/Zip:______________________________
____
Phone:______________________________
Fax:______________________________

SPECIALIST: ______________________________
Address:______________________________
____
City/State/Zip:______________________________
____
Phone:______________________________
Fax:______________________________

SPECIALIST: ______________________________
Address:______________________________
____
City/State/Zip:______________________________
____
Phone:______________________________
Fax:______________________________

SPECIALIST: ______________________________
Address:______________________________
____
City/State/Zip:______________________________
____
Phone:______________________________
Fax:______________________________

_______________Medications

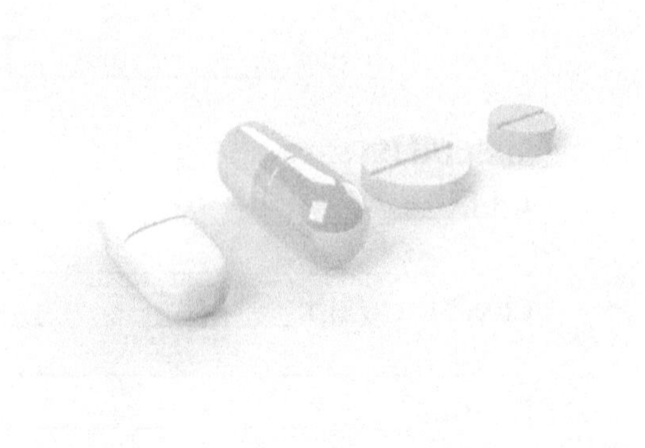

Prescriptions

Name	Dosage	Frequency	What's it For?

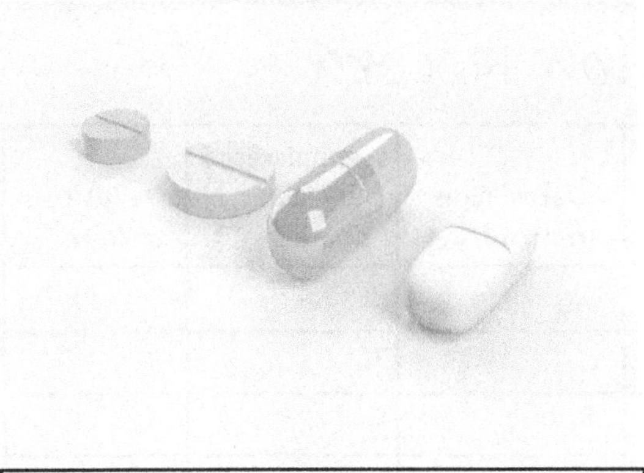

Vitamins and Supplements

Name	Dosage	Frequency	What's it For?

____________ Immunization Record

Vaccine	Type	Date Given (mm/dd/yy)	Administered by (clinic, doctor, etc)	Next Dose Date
Hepatitis B				
Rotavirus				
Diptheria, Tetanus, Pertusis (e.g. Tdap, Td)				
Haemophilus influenzae type b (Hib)				
Pneumococcal conjugate				
Inactivated poliovirus				

Immunization Record (cont'd)

Vaccine	Type	Date Given (mm/dd/yy)	Administered by (clinic, doctor, etc)	Next Dose Date
Influenza				
Measles, Mumps, Rubella				
Varicella (Checkenpox)				

________________ Immunization Record

Vaccine	Type	Date Given (mm/dd/yy)	Administered by (clinic, doctor, etc)	Next Dose Date
Hepatitis A				
Meningococcal ACWY				
Tetanus, diptheria, & acellular pertussis				
Human Pappilomavirus				
Meningococcal B				
Pneumococcal polysacharide				

How to Complete this Record

1. With the exception of hepatitis B vaccines, record the generic abbreviation (e.g., Tdap) or

   the trade name for each vaccine; for hepatitis B vaccines, record the trade name .
2. Record the type of vaccine (i.e. HepA-HepB)
3. Record the date given.
4. Record the source of the vaccine given (clinic, doctor, etc.).
5. Record when the next dose is due if necessary.

Immunization Record (cont'd)

Immunization information:

Diphtheria, tetanus, and pertussis (DTaP)

Routine vacc: 5-dose series at 2, 4, 6, 15-18 months, 4-6 years

Haemophilus influenzae type b vaccination

Routine vacc:

ActHIB, Hiberix, or Pentacel: 4-dose series at 2, 4, 6, 12-15 mos

PedvaxHIB: 3-dose series at 2, 4, 12-15 months

Hepatitis A

Routine vacc:—2-dose series

Hepatitis B

Routine vacc: 3 dose series at 0, 1-2, 6-18 months

Human papillomavirus vaccination

2– or 3-dose series depending on age at initial vaccination

Inactivated poliovirus vaccination

Routine vacc: 4-dose series at ages 2, 4, 6-18 mos, 4-6 yrs

Influenza vaccination

Routine vacc: 1 dose any influenza vaccine - annually

Measles, mumps, and rubella

Routine vacc: 2-dose series at 12-15 months, 4-6 years

Meningococcal ACWY

Routine vacc: 2-dose series: 11-12 years, 16 years

Pneumococcal vaccination

Routine vacc: 4-dose series at 2, 4, 6, 12-15 months

Rotavirus vaccination

Routine vacc:

Rotarix: 2-dose series at 2 and 4 months

RotaTeq: 3-dose series at 2, 4, and 6 months

Tetanus, diphtheria, and pertussis (Tdap) vaccination

Routine vaccination: Adolescents age 11-12 years—1 dose Tdap

Varicella vaccination

Routine vaccination: 2-dose series: 12-15 months, 4-6 years

______________ Medical Info

Blood Type: ______________________________

Allergies: ____

____

____

____

Medical Alert Information: ____

____

____

____

____

Previous Surgeries:

Date: ____________________ **Surgeon:** ______________________________________

Surgery: ____

____

____

Date: ____________________ **Surgeon:** ______________________________________

Surgery: ____

____

____

Date: ____________________ **Surgeon:** ______________________________________

Surgery: ____

____

____

Date: ____________________ **Surgeon:** ______________________________________

Surgery: ____

____

____

Date: ____________________ **Surgeon:** ______________________________________

Surgery: ____

____

____

Serious Injuries:

Date: ____________________ **Surgeon:** ____

Injury: ____

____

____

Date: ____________________ **Surgeon:** ____

Injury: ____

____

____

Date: ____________________ **Surgeon:** ____

Injury: ____

____

____

Date: ____________________ **Surgeon:** ____

Injury: ____

____

____

Date: ____________________ **Surgeon:** ____

Injury: ____

____

____

NOTES:

____________ Personal Medical History

	Rheumatic Fever		Lung (Pulmonary Disease)
	Heart Disease		COPD
	Heart Attack >50		Water on the Lungs
	Heart Attack <50		Asthma
	High Blood Pressure		Type I Diabetes
	AFib—Atrial Fibrillation		Type II Diabetes
	Pacemaker		Type III Diabetes
	Heart Murmur		Hepatitis A, B, or C
	High Cholesterol		Headaches/Migraines (w/aura)
	Stroke		Headaches/Migraines (w/out aura)
	Whooping Cough (Pertussis)		Seizure Disorder
	Measles		Epilepsy
	Meningitis		Digestive Tract
	Chicken Pox (Varicella)		Gallbladder/Gallstones
	Mumps		Diabetes
	Pneumonia		Liver Disease / Hepatitis
	Polio		Thyroid
	Tuberculosis		Kidney Renal Disease
	HIV Infection		Kidney Stones
	Eczema		Prostate Problems
	Tattoo		Rheumatoid Arthritis
	Hay Fever		Prior Orthopedic Problems
	Hives (Uticaria)		Joint Problems
	Allergies		Depression / Suicide
	Ear/Nose/Throat		Alcoholism
	Hearing Problems		Drug Addiction
	Immune Disorder		Anxiety

____________ Personal Medical History (cont'd)

	Skin Cancer		Panic Attacks
	Cancer		Mental Health Disorder
	Anemia		Fertility
	Hernia: Type ______________		Colon Polyps? ____
			Type: __________________

____________ Family Medical History

Condition	* G/A/U C/P/S	Condition	* G/A/U C/P/S
Heart Disease		Cancer	
Heart Attack		Breast	
High Blood Pressure		Colorectal	
High Cholesterol		Lung	
Kidney Disease		Prostate / Ovarian	
Lung Disease		Skin	
Asthma		Other: ____________	
COPD		Liver Disease	
Migraines		Stroke	
Dementia		Tuberculosis	
Alzheimers		Depression/Suicide	
Mental Disorder		Epilepsy/Seizures	
Thyroid Disease		Diabetes	
Smokers		Alcoholism	
Osteoporosis		Drug Addiction	

*** G/A/U/C/P/S = Grandparent, Aunt, Uncle, Cousin, Parent, Sibling**

________Doctors and Hospitals

HOSPITAL: ____________________
Address:____________________
____
City/State/Zip:____________________
____
Phone:____________________
Fax:____________________

PRIMARY CARE: ____________________
Address:____________________
____
City/State/Zip:____________________
____
Phone:____________________
Fax:____________________

DENTIST: ____________________
Address:____________________
____
City/State/Zip:____________________
____
Phone:____________________
Fax:____________________

OPTOMETRIST: ____________________
Address:____________________
____
City/State/Zip:____________________
____
Phone:____________________
Fax:____________________

SPECIALIST: ____________________
Address:____________________
____
City/State/Zip:____________________
____
Phone:____________________
Fax:____________________

________Doctors and Hospitals

SPECIALIST: ____
Address:____
____
City/State/Zip:____
____
Phone:____
Fax:____

SPECIALIST: ____
Address:____
____
City/State/Zip:____
____
Phone:____
Fax:____

SPECIALIST: ____
Address:____
____
City/State/Zip:____
____
Phone:____
Fax:____

SPECIALIST: ____
Address:____
____
City/State/Zip:____
____
Phone:____
Fax:____

SPECIALIST: ____
Address:____
____
City/State/Zip:____
____
Phone:____
Fax:____

____________Medications

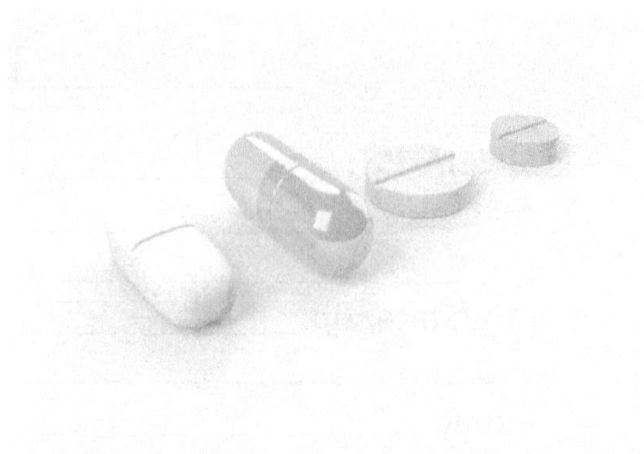

Prescriptions

Name	Dosage	Frequency	What's it For?

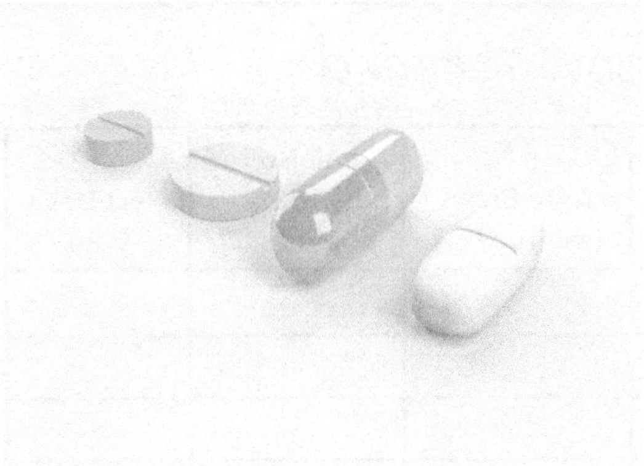

Vitamins and Supplements

Name	Dosage	Frequency	What's it For?

____________ Immunization Record

Vaccine	Type	Date Given (mm/dd/yy)	Administered by (clinic, doctor, etc)	Next Dose Date
Hepatitis B				
Rotavirus				
Diptheria, Tetanus, Pertusis (e.g. Tdap, Td)				
Haemophilus influenzae type b (Hib)				
Pneumococcal conjugate				
Inactivated poliovirus				

Immunization Record (cont'd)

Vaccine	Type	Date Given (mm/dd/yy)	Administered by (clinic, doctor, etc)	Next Dose Date
Influenza				
Measles, Mumps, Rubella				
Varicella (Checkenpox)				

______________ Immunization Record

Vaccine	Type	Date Given (mm/dd/yy)	Administered by (clinic, doctor, etc)	Next Dose Date
Hepatitis A				
Meningococcal ACWY				
Tetanus, diptheria, & acellular pertussis				
Human Pappilomavirus				
Meningococcal B				
Pneumococcal polysacharide				

How to Complete this Record

1. With the exception of hepatitis B vaccines, record the generic abbreviation (e.g., Tdap) or

   the trade name for each vaccine; for hepatitis B vaccines, record the trade name .
2. Record the type of vaccine (i.e. HepA-HepB)
3. Record the date given.
4. Record the source of the vaccine given (clinic, doctor, etc.).
5. Record when the next dose is due if necessary.

Immunization Record (cont'd)

Immunization information:

Diphtheria, tetanus, and pertussis (DTaP)

Routine vacc: 5-dose series at 2, 4, 6, 15-18 months, 4-6 years

Haemophilus influenzae type b vaccination

Routine vacc:

ActHIB, Hiberix, or Pentacel: 4-dose series at 2, 4, 6, 12-15 mos

PedvaxHIB: 3-dose series at 2, 4, 12-15 months

Hepatitis A

Routine vacc:—2-dose series

Hepatitis B

Routine vacc: 3 dose series at 0, 1-2, 6-18 months

Human papillomavirus vaccination

2– or 3-dose series depending on age at initial vaccination

Inactivated poliovirus vaccination

Routine vacc: 4-dose series at ages 2, 4, 6-18 mos, 4-6 yrs

Influenza vaccination

Routine vacc: 1 dose any influenza vaccine - annually

Measles, mumps, and rubella

Routine vacc: 2-dose series at 12-15 months, 4-6 years

Meningococcal ACWY

Routine vacc: 2-dose series: 11-12 years, 16 years

Pneumococcal vaccination

Routine vacc: 4-dose series at 2, 4, 6, 12-15 months

Rotavirus vaccination

Routine vacc:

Rotarix: 2-dose series at 2 and 4 months

RotaTeq: 3-dose series at 2, 4, and 6 months

Tetanus, diphtheria, and pertussis (Tdap) vaccination

Routine vaccination: Adolescents age 11-12 years—1 dose Tdap

Varicella vaccination

Routine vaccination: 2-dose series: 12-15 months, 4-6 years

________________ Medical Info

Blood Type: ____________________

Allergies: ____
____
____
____

Medical Alert Information: ____
____
____
____
____

Previous Surgeries:

Date: ______________ **Surgeon:** ______________________
Surgery: ____
____
____

Date: ______________ **Surgeon:** ______________________
Surgery: ____
____
____

Date: ______________ **Surgeon:** ______________________
Surgery: ____
____
____

Date: ______________ **Surgeon:** ______________________
Surgery: ____
____
____

Date: ______________ **Surgeon:** ______________________
Surgery: ____
____
____

Serious Injuries:

Date: ____________________ Surgeon: ____

Injury: ____

____

____

Date: ____________________ Surgeon: ____

Injury: ____

____

____

Date: ____________________ Surgeon: ____

Injury: ____

____

____

Date: ____________________ Surgeon: ____

Injury: ____

____

____

Date: ____________________ Surgeon: ____

Injury: ____

____

____

NOTES:

____________ Personal Medical History

	Rheumatic Fever		Lung (Pulmonary Disease)
	Heart Disease		COPD
	Heart Attack >50		Water on the Lungs
	Heart Attack <50		Asthma
	High Blood Pressure		Type I Diabetes
	AFib—Atrial Fibrillation		Type II Diabetes
	Pacemaker		Type III Diabetes
	Heart Murmur		Hepatitis A, B, or C
	High Cholesterol		Headaches/Migraines (w/aura)
	Stroke		Headaches/Migraines (w/out aura)
	Whooping Cough (Pertussis)		Seizure Disorder
	Measles		Epilepsy
	Meningitis		Digestive Tract
	Chicken Pox (Varicella)		Gallbladder/Gallstones
	Mumps		Diabetes
	Pneumonia		Liver Disease / Hepatitis
	Polio		Thyroid
	Tuberculosis		Kidney Renal Disease
	HIV Infection		Kidney Stones
	Eczema		Prostate Problems
	Tattoo		Rheumatoid Arthritis
	Hay Fever		Prior Orthopedic Problems
	Hives (Uticaria)		Joint Problems
	Allergies		Depression / Suicide
	Ear/Nose/Throat		Alcoholism
	Hearing Problems		Drug Addiction
	Immune Disorder		Anxiety

____________ Personal Medical History (cont'd)

	Skin Cancer		Panic Attacks
	Cancer		Mental Health Disorder
	Anemia		Fertility
	Hernia: Type ______________		Colon Polyps? ____
			Type: __________________

____________ Family Medical History

Condition	* G/A/U C/P/S	Condition	* G/A/U C/P/S
Heart Disease		Cancer	
Heart Attack		Breast	
High Blood Pressure		Colorectal	
High Cholesterol		Lung	
Kidney Disease		Prostate / Ovarian	
Lung Disease		Skin	
Asthma		Other: ____________	
COPD		Liver Disease	
Migraines		Stroke	
Dementia		Tuberculosis	
Alzheimers		Depression/Suicide	
Mental Disorder		Epilepsy/Seizures	
Thyroid Disease		Diabetes	
Smokers		Alcoholism	
Osteoporosis		Drug Addiction	

*** G/A/U/C/P/S = Grandparent, Aunt, Uncle, Cousin, Parent, Sibling**

________Doctors and Hospitals

HOSPITAL: ____
Address:____
____
City/State/Zip:____
____
Phone:____
Fax:____

PRIMARY CARE: ____
Address:____
____
City/State/Zip:____
____
Phone:____
Fax:____

DENTIST: ____
Address:____
____
City/State/Zip:____
____
Phone:____
Fax:____

OPTOMETRIST: ____
Address:____
____
City/State/Zip:____
____
Phone:____
Fax:____

SPECIALIST: ____
Address:____
____
City/State/Zip:____
____
Phone:____
Fax:____

________Doctors and Hospitals

SPECIALIST: ____________________
Address:____________________
____
City/State/Zip:____________________
____
Phone:____________________
Fax:____________________

SPECIALIST: ____________________
Address:____________________
____
City/State/Zip:____________________
____
Phone:____________________
Fax:____________________

SPECIALIST: ____________________
Address:____________________
____
City/State/Zip:____________________
____
Phone:____________________
Fax:____________________

SPECIALIST: ____________________
Address:____________________
____
City/State/Zip:____________________
____
Phone:____________________
Fax:____________________

SPECIALIST: ____________________
Address:____________________
____
City/State/Zip:____________________
____
Phone:____________________
Fax:____________________

______________Medications

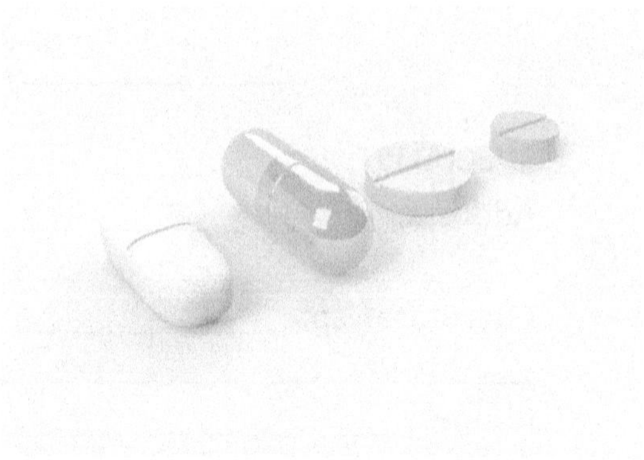

Prescriptions

Name	Dosage	Frequency	What's it For?

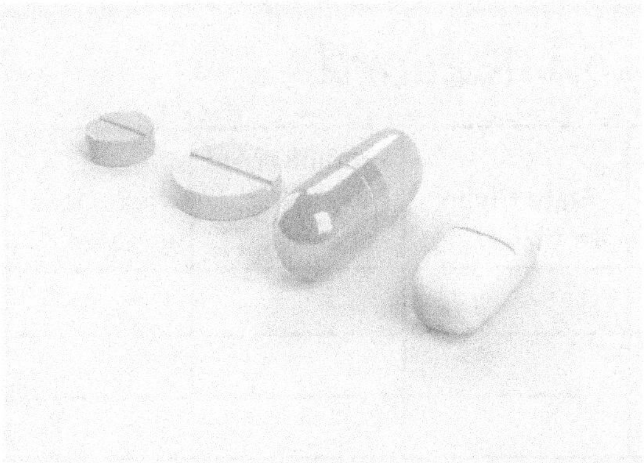

Vitamins and Supplements

Name	Dosage	Frequency	What's it For?

______________ Immunization Record

Vaccine	Type	Date Given (mm/dd/yy)	Administered by (clinic, doctor, etc)	Next Dose Date
Hepatitis B				
Rotavirus				
Diptheria, Tetanus, Pertusis (e.g. Tdap, Td)				
Haemophilus influenzae type b (Hib)				
Pneumococcal conjugate				
Inactivated poliovirus				

Immunization Record (cont'd)

Vaccine	Type	Date Given (mm/dd/yy)	Administered by (clinic, doctor, etc)	Next Dose Date
Influenza				
Measles, Mumps, Rubella				
Varicella (Checkenpox)				

____________ Immunization Record

Vaccine	Type	Date Given (mm/dd/yy)	Administered by (clinic, doctor, etc)	Next Dose Date
Hepatitis A				
Meningococcal ACWY				
Tetanus, diptheria, & acellular pertussis				
Human Pappilomavirus				
Meningococcal B				
Pneumococcal polysacharide				

How to Complete this Record

1. With the exception of hepatitis B vaccines, record the generic abbreviation (e.g., Tdap) or

   the trade name for each vaccine; for hepatitis B vaccines, record the trade name .
2. Record the type of vaccine (i.e. HepA-HepB)
3. Record the date given.
4. Record the source of the vaccine given (clinic, doctor, etc.).
5. Record when the next dose is due if necessary.

Immunization Record (cont'd)

Immunization information:

Diphtheria, tetanus, and pertussis (DTaP)

Routine vacc: 5-dose series at 2, 4, 6, 15-18 months, 4-6 years

Haemophilus influenzae type b vaccination

Routine vacc:

ActHIB, Hiberix, or Pentacel: 4-dose series at 2, 4, 6, 12-15 mos

PedvaxHIB: 3-dose series at 2, 4, 12-15 months

Hepatitis A

Routine vacc:—2-dose series

Hepatitis B

Routine vacc: 3 dose series at 0, 1-2, 6-18 months

Human papillomavirus vaccination

2– or 3-dose series depending on age at initial vaccination

Inactivated poliovirus vaccination

Routine vacc: 4-dose series at ages 2, 4, 6-18 mos, 4-6 yrs

Influenza vaccination

Routine vacc: 1 dose any influenza vaccine - annually

Measles, mumps, and rubella

Routine vacc: 2-dose series at 12-15 months, 4-6 years

Meningococcal ACWY

Routine vacc: 2-dose series: 11-12 years, 16 years

Pneumococcal vaccination

Routine vacc: 4-dose series at 2, 4, 6, 12-15 months

Rotavirus vaccination

Routine vacc:

Rotarix: 2-dose series at 2 and 4 months

RotaTeq: 3-dose series at 2, 4, and 6 months

Tetanus, diphtheria, and pertussis (Tdap) vaccination

Routine vaccination: Adolescents age 11-12 years—1 dose Tdap

Varicella vaccination

Routine vaccination: 2-dose series: 12-15 months, 4-6 years

____________ Medical Info

Blood Type: ____________________

Allergies: ____

____

____

____

Medical Alert Information: ________________________________

____

____

____

____

Previous Surgeries:

Date: ______________ **Surgeon:** ____________________

Surgery: ____

____

____

Date: ______________ **Surgeon:** ____________________

Surgery: ____

____

____

Date: ______________ **Surgeon:** ____________________

Surgery: ____

____

____

Date: ______________ **Surgeon:** ____________________

Surgery: ____

____

____

Date: ______________ **Surgeon:** ____________________

Surgery: ____

____

____

Serious Injuries:

Date: ____________________ **Surgeon:** ____

Injury: ____

____

____

Date: ____________________ **Surgeon:** ____

Injury: ____

____

____

Date: ____________________ **Surgeon:** ____

Injury: ____

____

____

Date: ____________________ **Surgeon:** ____

Injury: ____

____

____

Date: ____________________ **Surgeon:** ____

Injury: ____

____

____

NOTES:

_____________ Personal Medical History

	Rheumatic Fever		Lung (Pulmonary Disease)
	Heart Disease		COPD
	Heart Attack >50		Water on the Lungs
	Heart Attack <50		Asthma
	High Blood Pressure		Type I Diabetes
	AFib—Atrial Fibrillation		Type II Diabetes
	Pacemaker		Type III Diabetes
	Heart Murmur		Hepatitis A, B, or C
	High Cholesterol		Headaches/Migraines (w/aura)
	Stroke		Headaches/Migraines (w/out aura)
	Whooping Cough (Pertussis)		Seizure Disorder
	Measles		Epilepsy
	Meningitis		Digestive Tract
	Chicken Pox (Varicella)		Gallbladder/Gallstones
	Mumps		Diabetes
	Pneumonia		Liver Disease / Hepatitis
	Polio		Thyroid
	Tuberculosis		Kidney Renal Disease
	HIV Infection		Kidney Stones
	Eczema		Prostate Problems
	Tattoo		Rheumatoid Arthritis
	Hay Fever		Prior Orthopedic Problems
	Hives (Uticaria)		Joint Problems
	Allergies		Depression / Suicide
	Ear/Nose/Throat		Alcoholism
	Hearing Problems		Drug Addiction
	Immune Disorder		Anxiety

____________ Personal Medical History (cont'd)

	Skin Cancer		Panic Attacks
	Cancer		Mental Health Disorder
	Anemia		Fertility
	Hernia: Type ______________		Colon Polyps? ____
			Type: __________________

____________ Family Medical History

Condition	* G/A/U C/P/S	Condition	* G/A/U C/P/S
Heart Disease		Cancer	
Heart Attack		Breast	
High Blood Pressure		Colorectal	
High Cholesterol		Lung	
Kidney Disease		Prostate / Ovarian	
Lung Disease		Skin	
Asthma		Other: ____________	
COPD		Liver Disease	
Migraines		Stroke	
Dementia		Tuberculosis	
Alzheimers		Depression/Suicide	
Mental Disorder		Epilepsy/Seizures	
Thyroid Disease		Diabetes	
Smokers		Alcoholism	
Osteoporosis		Drug Addiction	

*** G/A/U/C/P/S = Grandparent, Aunt, Uncle, Cousin, Parent, Sibling**

________Doctors and Hospitals

HOSPITAL: ______________________________________
Address:______________________________________
____
City/State/Zip:______________________________________
____
Phone:______________________________________
Fax:______________________________________

PRIMARY CARE: ______________________________________
Address:______________________________________
____
City/State/Zip:______________________________________
____
Phone:______________________________________
Fax:______________________________________

DENTIST: ______________________________________
Address:______________________________________
____
City/State/Zip:______________________________________
____
Phone:______________________________________
Fax:______________________________________

OPTOMETRIST: ______________________________________
Address:______________________________________
____
City/State/Zip:______________________________________
____
Phone:______________________________________
Fax:______________________________________

SPECIALIST: ______________________________________
Address:______________________________________
____
City/State/Zip:______________________________________
____
Phone:______________________________________
Fax:______________________________________

________Doctors and Hospitals

SPECIALIST: ____________________
Address:____________________
____
City/State/Zip:____________________
____
Phone:____________________
Fax:____________________

SPECIALIST: ____________________
Address:____________________
____
City/State/Zip:____________________
____
Phone:____________________
Fax:____________________

SPECIALIST: ____________________
Address:____________________
____
City/State/Zip:____________________
____
Phone:____________________
Fax:____________________

SPECIALIST: ____________________
Address:____________________
____
City/State/Zip:____________________
____
Phone:____________________
Fax:____________________

SPECIALIST: ____________________
Address:____________________
____
City/State/Zip:____________________
____
Phone:____________________
Fax:____________________

____________Medications

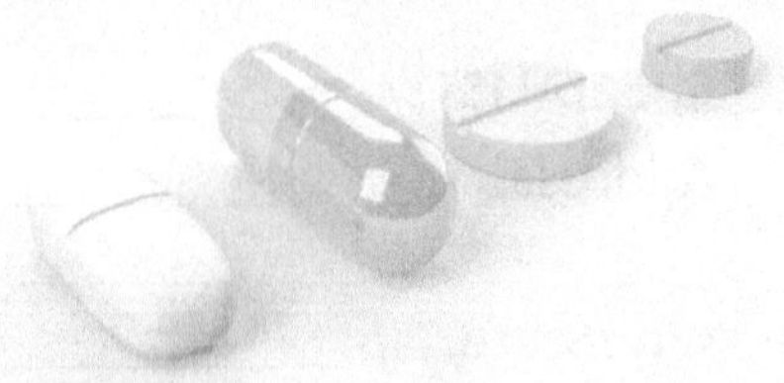

Prescriptions

Name	Dosage	Frequency	What's it For?

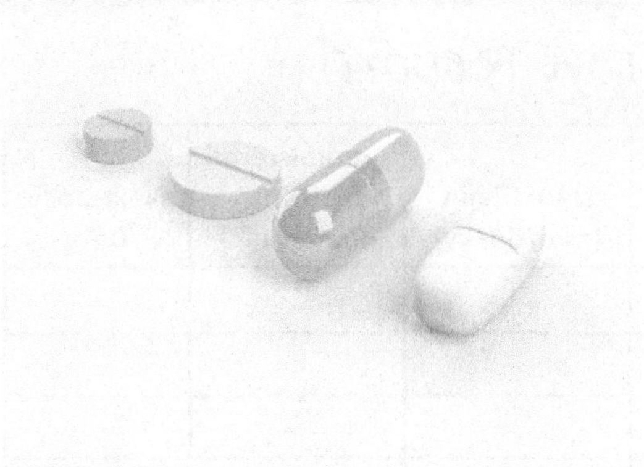

Vitamins and Supplements

Name	Dosage	Frequency	What's it For?

____________ Immunization Record

Vaccine	Type	Date Given (mm/dd/yy)	Administered by (clinic, doctor, etc)	Next Dose Date
Hepatitis B				
Rotavirus				
Diptheria, Tetanus, Pertusis (e.g. Tdap, Td)				
Haemophilus influenzae type b (Hib)				
Pneumococcal conjugate				
Inactivated poliovirus				

Immunization Record (cont'd)

Vaccine	Type	Date Given (mm/dd/yy)	Administered by (clinic, doctor, etc)	Next Dose Date
Influenza				
Measles, Mumps, Rubella				
Varicella (Checkenpox)				

_______________ Immunization Record

Vaccine	Type	Date Given (mm/dd/yy)	Administered by (clinic, doctor, etc)	Next Dose Date
Hepatitis A				
Meningococcal ACWY				
Tetanus, diptheria, & acellular pertussis				
Human Pappilomavirus				
Meningococcal B				
Pneumococcal polysacharide				

How to Complete this Record

1. With the exception of hepatitis B vaccines, record the generic abbreviation (e.g., Tdap) or

   the trade name for each vaccine; for hepatitis B vaccines, record the trade name .
2. Record the type of vaccine (i.e. HepA-HepB)
3. Record the date given.
4. Record the source of the vaccine given (clinic, doctor, etc.).
5. Record when the next dose is due if necessary.

Immunization Record (cont'd)

Immunization information:

Diphtheria, tetanus, and pertussis (DTaP)

Routine vacc: 5-dose series at 2, 4, 6, 15-18 months, 4-6 years

Haemophilus influenzae type b vaccination

Routine vacc:

ActHIB, Hiberix, or Pentacel: 4-dose series at 2, 4, 6, 12-15 mos

PedvaxHIB: 3-dose series at 2, 4, 12-15 months

Hepatitis A

Routine vacc:—2-dose series

Hepatitis B

Routine vacc: 3 dose series at 0, 1-2, 6-18 months

Human papillomavirus vaccination

2– or 3-dose series depending on age at initial vaccination

Inactivated poliovirus vaccination

Routine vacc: 4-dose series at ages 2, 4, 6-18 mos, 4-6 yrs

Influenza vaccination

Routine vacc: 1 dose any influenza vaccine - annually

Measles, mumps, and rubella

Routine vacc: 2-dose series at 12-15 months, 4-6 years

Meningococcal ACWY

Routine vacc: 2-dose series: 11-12 years, 16 years

Pneumococcal vaccination

Routine vacc: 4-dose series at 2, 4, 6, 12-15 months

Rotavirus vaccination

Routine vacc:

Rotarix: 2-dose series at 2 and 4 months

RotaTeq: 3-dose series at 2, 4, and 6 months

Tetanus, diphtheria, and pertussis (Tdap) vaccination

Routine vaccination: Adolescents age 11-12 years—1 dose Tdap

Varicella vaccination

Routine vaccination: 2-dose series: 12-15 months, 4-6 years

Office Visit

For ______________________________

Date/Time: ______________________________

Name: ______________________________

Doctor: ______________________________

Reason for Visit: ______________________________

____

____

____

____

Questions to ask the doctor: ______________________________

____

____

____

____

____

____

____

____

____

Doctor's Diagnosis/Feedback: ______________________________

____

____

____

____

____

____

____

____

____

Weight ____________________ **Blood Pressure** ____________________

Temperature ____________________ **Heart Rate** ____________________

Office Visit

Is a follow-up visit needed? ________

Date for next visit: ______________________________

Tests Ordered	Test Results

Treatment Received Today:____

____

____

____

Any medication changes?

____

____

____

NOTES

Office Visit

For ______________________________

Date/Time: ______________________________

Name: ______________________________

Doctor: ______________________________

Reason for Visit: ______________________________

____

____

____

____

Questions to ask the doctor: ______________________________

____

____

____

____

____

____

____

____

____

Doctor's Diagnosis/Feedback: ______________________________

____

____

____

____

____

____

____

____

____

Weight ____________________ **Blood Pressure** ____________________

Temperature ____________________ **Heart Rate** ____________________

Office Visit

Is a follow-up visit needed? ________

Date for next visit: ______________________________

Tests Ordered	Test Results

Treatment Received Today:____
____
____
____

Any medication changes?

____
____
____

NOTES

Office Visit

For ______________________________

Date/Time:______________________________

Name:______________________________

Doctor:______________________________

Reason for Visit:______________________________

____

____

____

____

Questions to ask the doctor:______________________________

____

____

____

____

____

____

____

____

____

Doctor's Diagnosis/Feedback: ______________________________

____

____

____

____

____

____

____

____

____

Weight______________________ **Blood Pressure**______________________

Temperature______________________ **Heart Rate**______________________

Office Visit

Is a follow-up visit needed? ________

Date for next visit: ____________________________

Tests Ordered	Test Results

Treatment Received Today:____

____

____

____

Any medication changes?

____

____

____

NOTES

Office Visit

For ______________________________

Date/Time: ______________________________

Name: ______________________________

Doctor: ______________________________

Reason for Visit: ______________________________

____

____

____

____

Questions to ask the doctor: ______________________________

____

____

____

____

____

____

____

____

____

Doctor's Diagnosis/Feedback: ______________________________

____

____

____

____

____

____

____

____

____

Weight ____________________ **Blood Pressure** ____________________

Temperature ____________________ **Heart Rate** ____________________

Office Visit

Is a follow-up visit needed? ________

Date for next visit: ____________________________

Tests Ordered	Test Results

Treatment Received Today:____

____

____

____

Any medication changes?

____

____

____

NOTES

Office Visit

For ______________________________

Date/Time:____

Name:____

Doctor:____

Reason for Visit:____

____

____

____

____

Questions to ask the doctor:____

____

____

____

____

____

____

____

____

____

Doctor's Diagnosis/Feedback: ____

____

____

____

____

____

____

____

____

____

Weight______________________ **Blood Pressure**______________________

Temperature______________________ **Heart Rate**______________________

Office Visit

Is a follow-up visit needed? ________

Date for next visit: ______________________________

Tests Ordered	Test Results

Treatment Received Today:____

____

____

____

Any medication changes?

____

____

____

NOTES

Office Visit

For ______________________________

Date/Time:______________________________

Name:______________________________

Doctor:______________________________

Reason for Visit:______________________________

____

____

____

____

Questions to ask the doctor:______________________________

____

____

____

____

____

____

____

____

____

Doctor's Diagnosis/Feedback: ______________________________

____

____

____

____

____

____

____

____

____

Weight______________________ **Blood Pressure**______________________

Temperature______________________ **Heart Rate**______________________

Office Visit

Is a follow-up visit needed? ________

Date for next visit: ____________________________

Tests Ordered	Test Results

Treatment Received Today:____

____

____

____

Any medication changes?

____

____

____

NOTES

Office Visit

For ______________________________

Date/Time:______________________________

Name:______________________________

Doctor:______________________________

Reason for Visit:______________________________

____

____

____

____

Questions to ask the doctor:______________________________

____

____

____

____

____

____

____

____

____

Doctor's Diagnosis/Feedback: ______________________________

____

____

____

____

____

____

____

____

____

Weight______________________ **Blood Pressure**______________________

Temperature______________________ **Heart Rate**______________________

Office Visit

Is a follow-up visit needed? ________

Date for next visit: ______________________________

Tests Ordered	Test Results

Treatment Received Today:____

____

____

____

Any medication changes?

____

____

____

NOTES

Office Visit

For ________________________________

Date/Time:____

Name:____

Doctor:____

Reason for Visit:____

____

____

____

____

Questions to ask the doctor:____

____

____

____

____

____

____

____

____

____

Doctor's Diagnosis/Feedback: ____

____

____

____

____

____

____

____

____

____

Weight__________________________ **Blood Pressure**________________________

Temperature_____________________ **Heart Rate**____________________________

Office Visit

Is a follow-up visit needed? ________

Date for next visit: ______________________________

Tests Ordered	Test Results

Treatment Received Today:____
____
____
____

Any medication changes?

____
____
____

NOTES

Office Visit

For ______________________________

Date/Time: ______________________________

Name: ______________________________

Doctor: ______________________________

Reason for Visit: ______________________________

Questions to ask the doctor: ______________________________

Doctor's Diagnosis/Feedback: ______________________________

Weight ______________ Blood Pressure ______________

Temperature ______________ Heart Rate ______________

Office Visit

Is a follow-up visit needed? ________

Date for next visit: ______________________________

Tests Ordered	Test Results

Treatment Received Today:____

____

____

____

Any medication changes?

____

____

____

NOTES

Office Visit

For ______________________________

Date/Time: ______________________________

Name: ______________________________

Doctor: ______________________________

Reason for Visit: ______________________________

____

____

____

____

Questions to ask the doctor: ______________________________

____

____

____

____

____

____

____

____

____

Doctor's Diagnosis/Feedback: ______________________________

____

____

____

____

____

____

____

____

____

Weight ____________________ **Blood Pressure** ____________________

Temperature ____________________ **Heart Rate** ____________________

Office Visit

Is a follow-up visit needed? ________

Date for next visit: ______________________________

Tests Ordered	Test Results

Treatment Received Today:____

____

____

____

Any medication changes?

____

____

____

NOTES

Office Visit

For ______________________________

Date/Time:______________________________

Name:______________________________

Doctor:______________________________

Reason for Visit:______________________________

____

____

____

____

Questions to ask the doctor:______________________________

____

____

____

____

____

____

____

____

____

Doctor's Diagnosis/Feedback: ______________________________

____

____

____

____

____

____

____

____

____

Weight______________________ **Blood Pressure**______________________

Temperature______________________ **Heart Rate**______________________

Office Visit

Is a follow-up visit needed? ________

Date for next visit: ____________________________

Tests Ordered	Test Results

Treatment Received Today:____

____

____

____

Any medication changes?

____

____

____

NOTES

Office Visit

For ______________________________

Date/Time:______________________________

Name:______________________________

Doctor:______________________________

Reason for Visit:______________________________

____

____

____

____

Questions to ask the doctor:______________________________

____

____

____

____

____

____

____

____

____

Doctor's Diagnosis/Feedback: ______________________________

____

____

____

____

____

____

____

____

____

Weight____________________ **Blood Pressure**____________________

Temperature____________________ **Heart Rate**____________________

Office Visit

Is a follow-up visit needed? ________

Date for next visit: ______________________________

Tests Ordered	Test Results

Treatment Received Today:____

____

____

____

Any medication changes?

____

____

____

NOTES

Office Visit

For ______________________________

Date/Time:____

Name:____

Doctor:____

Reason for Visit:____

____

____

____

____

Questions to ask the doctor:____

____

____

____

____

____

____

____

____

____

Doctor's Diagnosis/Feedback: ____

____

____

____

____

____

____

____

____

____

Weight________________________ **Blood Pressure**______________________

Temperature____________________ **Heart Rate**_________________________

Office Visit

Is a follow-up visit needed? _________

Date for next visit: ______________________________

Tests Ordered	Test Results

Treatment Received Today:____

____

____

____

Any medication changes?

____

____

____

NOTES

Office Visit

For ______________________________

Date/Time:____

Name:____

Doctor:____

Reason for Visit:____

____

____

____

____

Questions to ask the doctor:____

____

____

____

____

____

____

____

____

____

Doctor's Diagnosis/Feedback: ____

____

____

____

____

____

____

____

____

____

Weight________________________ **Blood Pressure**______________________

Temperature___________________ **Heart Rate**__________________________

Office Visit

Is a follow-up visit needed? ________

Date for next visit: ______________________________

Tests Ordered	Test Results

Treatment Received Today:____

____

____

____

Any medication changes?

____

____

____

NOTES

Office Visit

For ______________________________

Date/Time: ______________________________

Name: ______________________________

Doctor: ______________________________

Reason for Visit: ______________________________

Questions to ask the doctor: ______________________________

Doctor's Diagnosis/Feedback: ______________________________

Weight ______________ **Blood Pressure** ______________

Temperature ______________ **Heart Rate** ______________

Office Visit

Is a follow-up visit needed? ________

Date for next visit: ______________________________

Tests Ordered	Test Results

Treatment Received Today:____

____

____

____

Any medication changes?

____

____

____

NOTES

Office Visit

For ________________________________

Date/Time:____

Name:____

Doctor:____

Reason for Visit:____

____

____

____

____

Questions to ask the doctor:____

____

____

____

____

____

____

____

____

____

Doctor's Diagnosis/Feedback: ____

____

____

____

____

____

____

____

____

____

Weight______________________ **Blood Pressure**______________________

Temperature______________________ **Heart Rate**______________________

Office Visit

Is a follow-up visit needed? ________

Date for next visit: ______________________________

Tests Ordered	Test Results

Treatment Received Today:____

____

____

____

Any medication changes?

____

____

____

NOTES

Office Visit

For ______________________

Date/Time: ______________________

Name: ______________________

Doctor: ______________________

Reason for Visit: ______________________

Questions to ask the doctor: ______________________

Doctor's Diagnosis/Feedback: ______________________

Weight ______________ **Blood Pressure** ______________

Temperature ______________ **Heart Rate** ______________

Office Visit

Is a follow-up visit needed? ________

Date for next visit: ______________________________

Tests Ordered	Test Results

Treatment Received Today:____
____
____
____

Any medication changes?

____
____
____

NOTES

Office Visit

For ______________________________

Date/Time: ______________________________

Name: ______________________________

Doctor: ______________________________

Reason for Visit: ______________________________

____

____

____

____

Questions to ask the doctor: ______________________________

____

____

____

____

____

____

____

____

____

Doctor's Diagnosis/Feedback: ______________________________

____

____

____

____

____

____

____

____

____

Weight ____________________ **Blood Pressure** ____________________

Temperature ____________________ **Heart Rate** ____________________

Office Visit

Is a follow-up visit needed? ________

Date for next visit: ____________________________

Tests Ordered	Test Results

Treatment Received Today:____

____

____

____

Any medication changes?

____

____

____

NOTES

Office Visit

For ______________________________

Date/Time:____

Name:____

Doctor:____

Reason for Visit:____

____

____

____

____

Questions to ask the doctor:____

____

____

____

____

____

____

____

____

____

Doctor's Diagnosis/Feedback: ____

____

____

____

____

____

____

____

____

____

Weight______________________ **Blood Pressure**______________________

Temperature______________________ **Heart Rate**______________________

Office Visit

Is a follow-up visit needed? _________

Date for next visit: _______________________________

Tests Ordered	Test Results

Treatment Received Today:____

____

____

____

Any medication changes?

____

____

____

NOTES

Office Visit

For ______________________________

Date/Time:______________________________

Name:______________________________

Doctor:______________________________

Reason for Visit:______________________________

____

____

____

____

Questions to ask the doctor:______________________________

____

____

____

____

____

____

____

____

____

Doctor's Diagnosis/Feedback: ______________________________

____

____

____

____

____

____

____

____

____

Weight______________________ **Blood Pressure**______________________

Temperature______________________ **Heart Rate**______________________

Office Visit

Is a follow-up visit needed? ________

Date for next visit: ______________________________

Tests Ordered	Test Results

Treatment Received Today:____
____
____
____

Any medication changes?

____
____
____

NOTES

Office Visit

For ______________________________

Date/Time:______________________________

Name:______________________________

Doctor:______________________________

Reason for Visit:______________________________

____

____

____

____

Questions to ask the doctor:______________________________

____

____

____

____

____

____

____

____

____

Doctor's Diagnosis/Feedback: ______________________________

____

____

____

____

____

____

____

____

____

Weight______________________ **Blood Pressure**______________________

Temperature______________________ **Heart Rate**______________________

Office Visit

Is a follow-up visit needed? ________

Date for next visit: ______________________________

Tests Ordered	Test Results

Treatment Received Today:____

____

____

____

Any medication changes?

____

____

____

NOTES

Office Visit

For ______________________________

Date/Time:______________________________

Name:______________________________

Doctor:______________________________

Reason for Visit:______________________________

____

____

____

____

Questions to ask the doctor:______________________________

____

____

____

____

____

____

____

____

____

Doctor's Diagnosis/Feedback: ______________________________

____

____

____

____

____

____

____

____

____

Weight______________________ **Blood Pressure**______________________

Temperature______________________ **Heart Rate**______________________

Office Visit

Is a follow-up visit needed? ________

Date for next visit: ____________________________

Tests Ordered	Test Results

Treatment Received Today:____

____

____

____

Any medication changes?

____

____

____

NOTES

Office Visit

For ______________________________

Date/Time:______________________________

Name:______________________________

Doctor:______________________________

Reason for Visit:______________________________

Questions to ask the doctor:______________________________

Doctor's Diagnosis/Feedback: ______________________________

Weight______________________ **Blood Pressure**______________________

Temperature______________________ **Heart Rate**______________________

Office Visit

Is a follow-up visit needed? ________

Date for next visit: ____________________________

Tests Ordered	Test Results

Treatment Received Today:____

____

____

____

Any medication changes?

____

____

____

NOTES

Office Visit

For ______________________________

Date/Time:______________________________

Name:______________________________

Doctor:______________________________

Reason for Visit:______________________________

Questions to ask the doctor:______________________________

Doctor's Diagnosis/Feedback: ______________________________

Weight____________________ **Blood Pressure**____________________

Temperature____________________ **Heart Rate**____________________

Office Visit

Is a follow-up visit needed? _________

Date for next visit: ______________________________

Tests Ordered	Test Results

Treatment Received Today:____

____

____

____

Any medication changes?

____

____

____

NOTES

Office Visit

For ______________________________

Date/Time:____

Name:____

Doctor:____

Reason for Visit:____

Questions to ask the doctor:____

Doctor's Diagnosis/Feedback: ____

Weight________________________ **Blood Pressure**______________________

Temperature____________________ **Heart Rate**_________________________

Office Visit

Is a follow-up visit needed? _________

Date for next visit: ______________________________

Tests Ordered	Test Results

Treatment Received Today:____
____
____
____

Any medication changes?

____
____
____

NOTES

Other books available by the author on Amazon

Go to Amazon.com and enter "Dianne Terry" in the search bar for more details for each of these books.

Journals

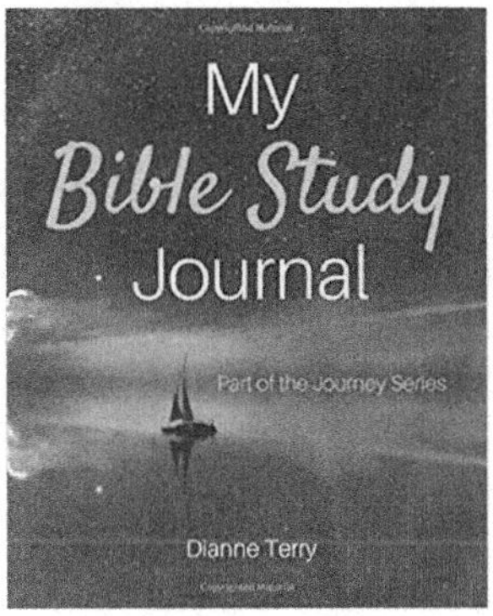

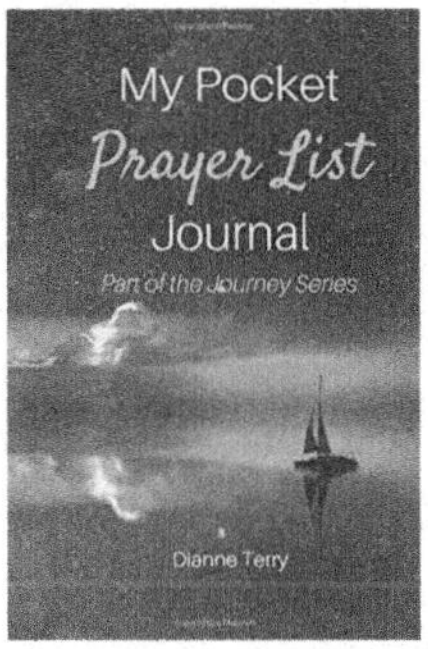

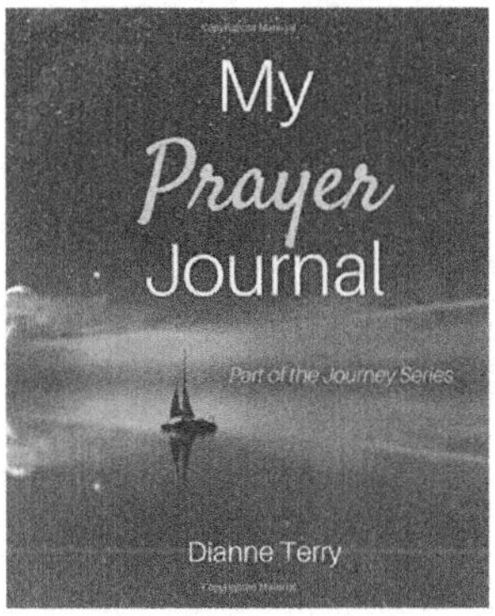

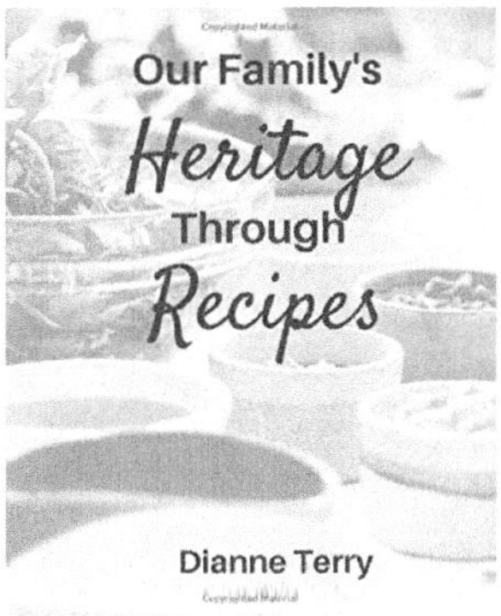

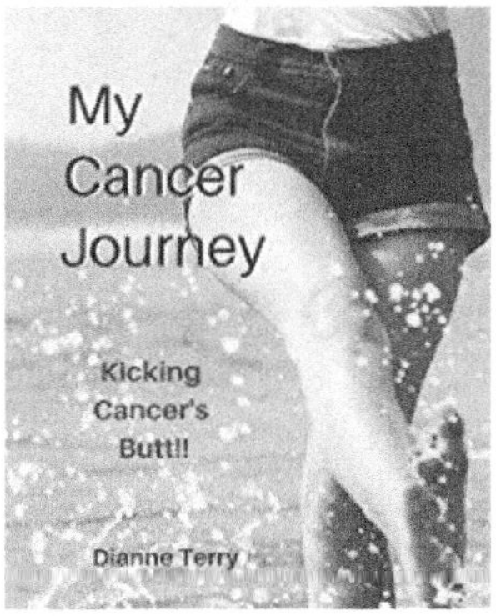

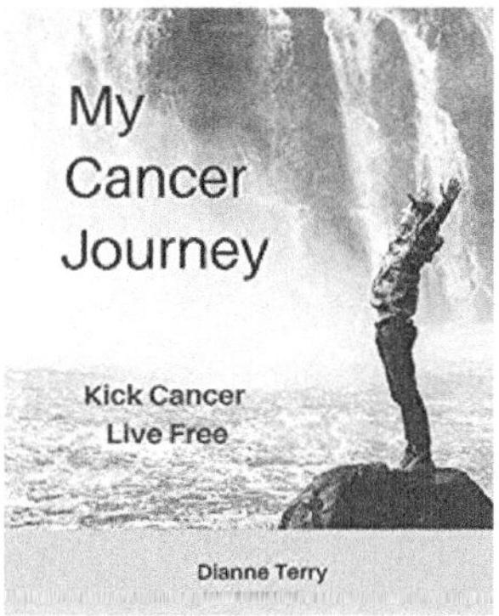

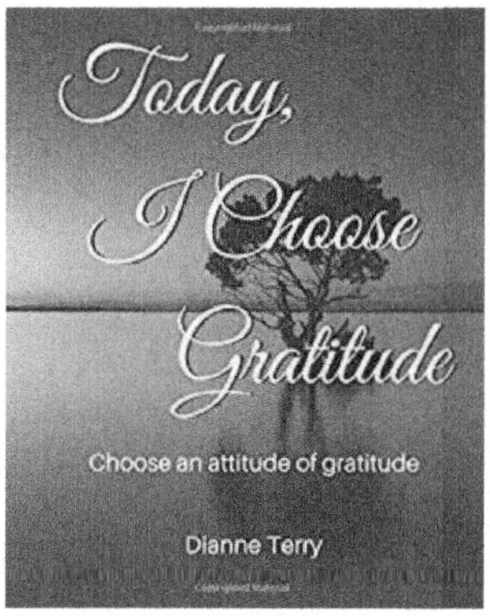

Gift Books

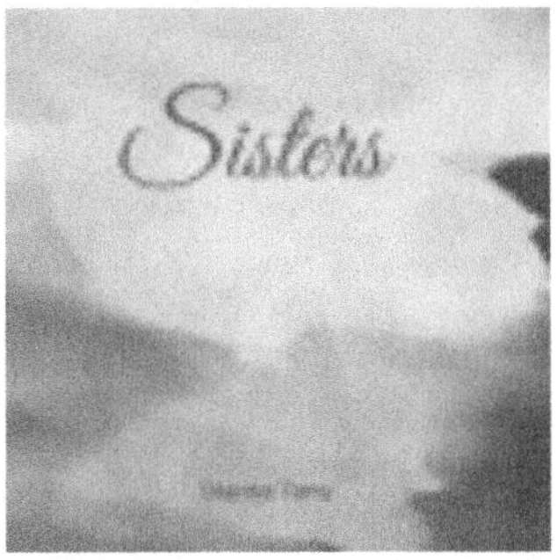

Made in the USA
Monee, IL
05 November 2026

67377177R00096